For everyone who's ever given me a chance. —Sofia Sanchez

For you. —Meg O'Hair

For those who are still learning how to
embrace what makes them one of a kind. —Sofia Cardoso

Text copyright © 2021 by Margaret O'Hair

Illustrations copyright © 2021 by Scholastic Inc.

Photo credits: © Jennifer Varanini Sanchez

Library of Congress Cataloging-in-Publication Data available

ISBN 978-1-338-63074-9

10 9 8 7 6 5 4 3 2 1   21 22 23 24 25

Printed in China   38

First edition, March 2021

Book design by Katie Fitch

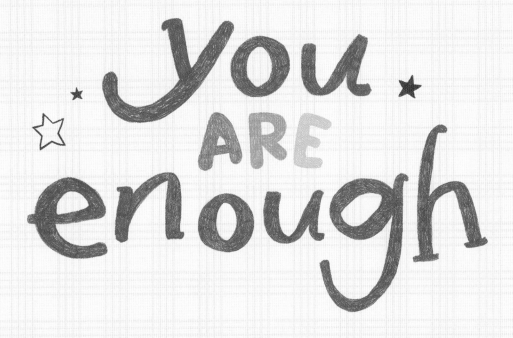

You ARE enough

A BOOK ABOUT INCLUSION

Inspired by
SOFIA SANCHEZ

Written by Margaret O'Hair   Illustrated by Sofia Cardoso

Scholastic Inc.

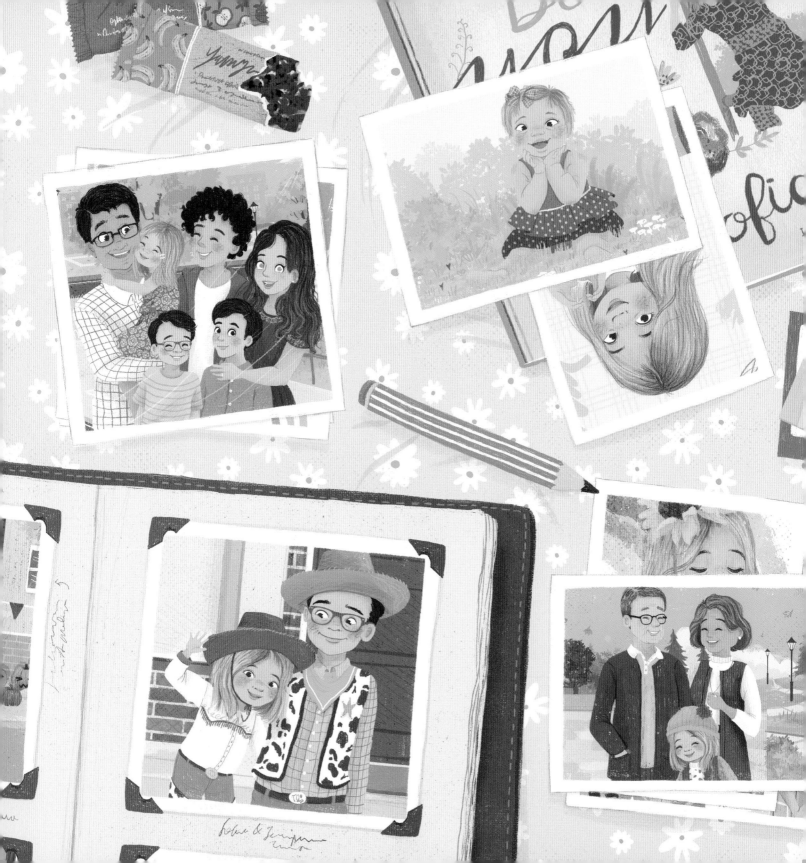

My name is Sofia Sanchez, and I have Down syndrome. That means I look and learn differently than most people. I was born in a small town in Ukraine, where I spent the first sixteen months of my life in an orphanage. But in June 2010, my forever mom and dad took me home to the United States, where I live with them and my three older brothers. One of my brothers has Down syndrome, too.

I am just like any other kid. I like to read and draw in my journal. I love people and making new friends. I dance and cheer, and my favorite subjects are Spanish, music, and theater. My mom and dad are always taking pictures and videos of me. I love the camera! That's how I began my acting and modeling career.

I am only a kid, but I know I am someone who is happy, loving, and kind. I have Down syndrome, and it makes some things harder for me, but it's just one part of who I am. I believe in myself. And I want to inspire others to love themselves, too. Because we are all beautiful, just as we are.

No two people are exactly the same.

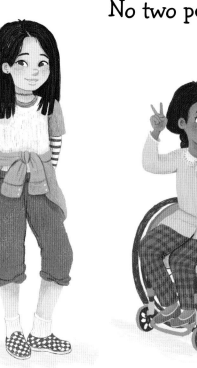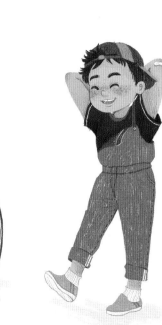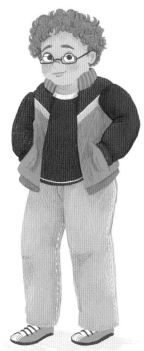

We are all unique—and that's great!

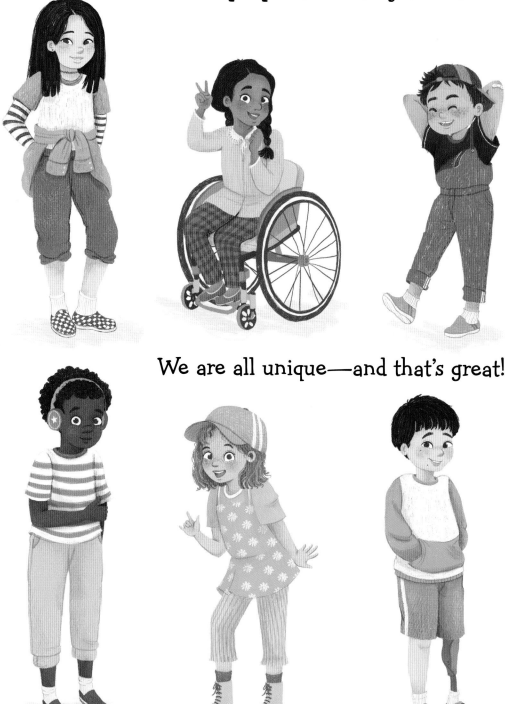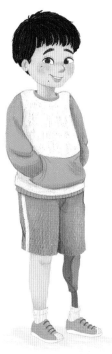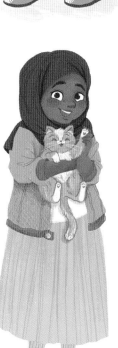

Being different is what makes you special.

You are just right exactly as you are.

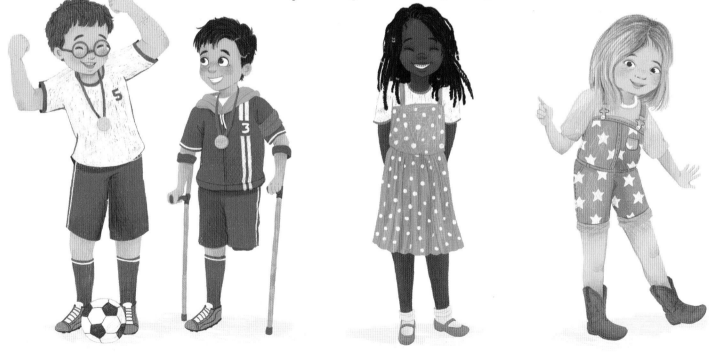

Being different can be lonely.

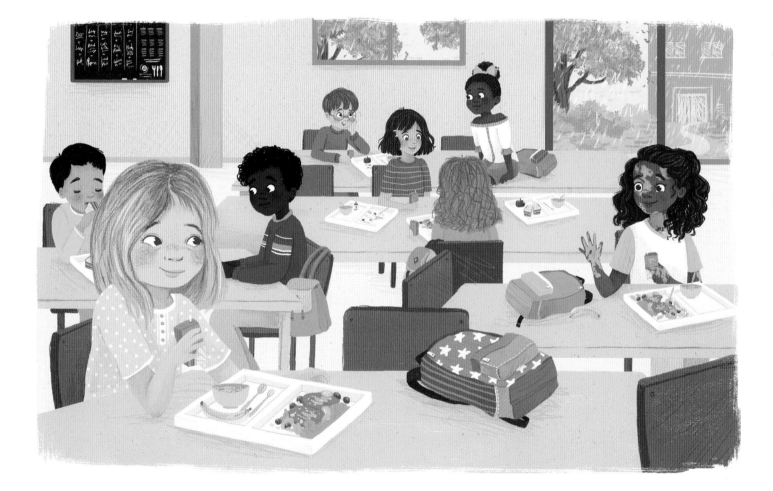

You may feel like you don't belong.

But we're all in this together.

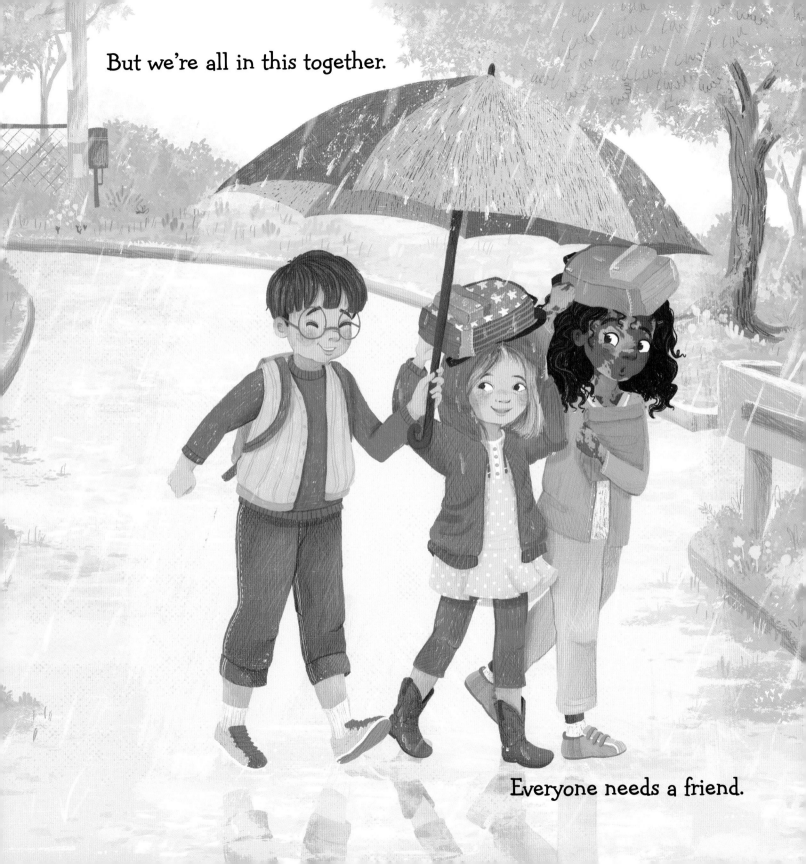

Everyone needs a friend.

Friends help one another.

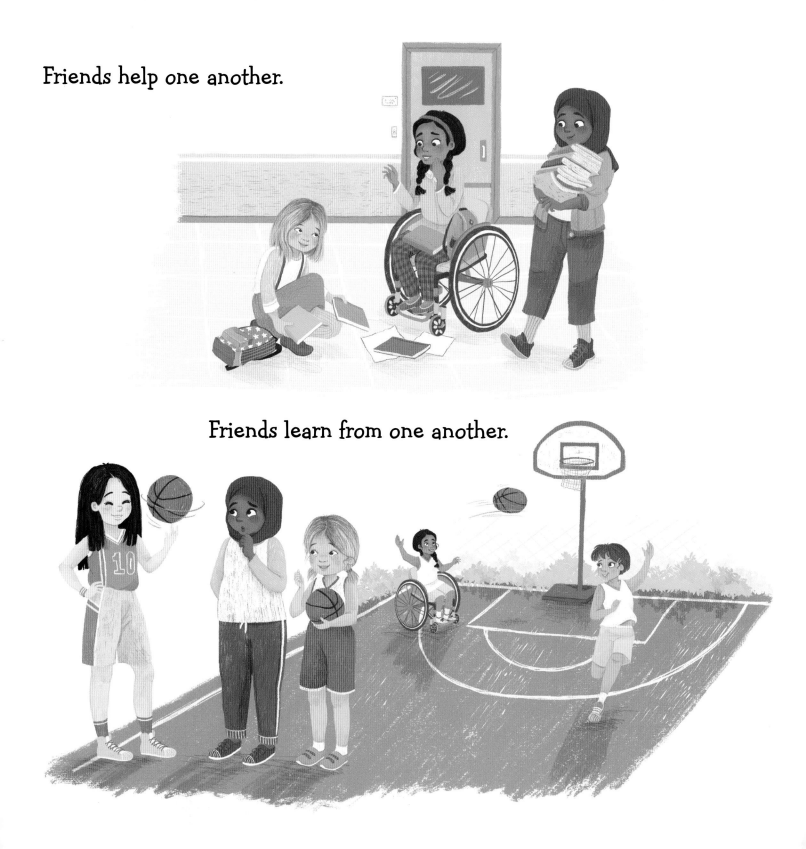

Friends learn from one another.

Friends know that no
two people are alike.

A friend will celebrate
YOU just as you are!

But some people don't understand.

They think being different is scary.

Don't stay on the sidelines.

It's YOUR story—so be the star!

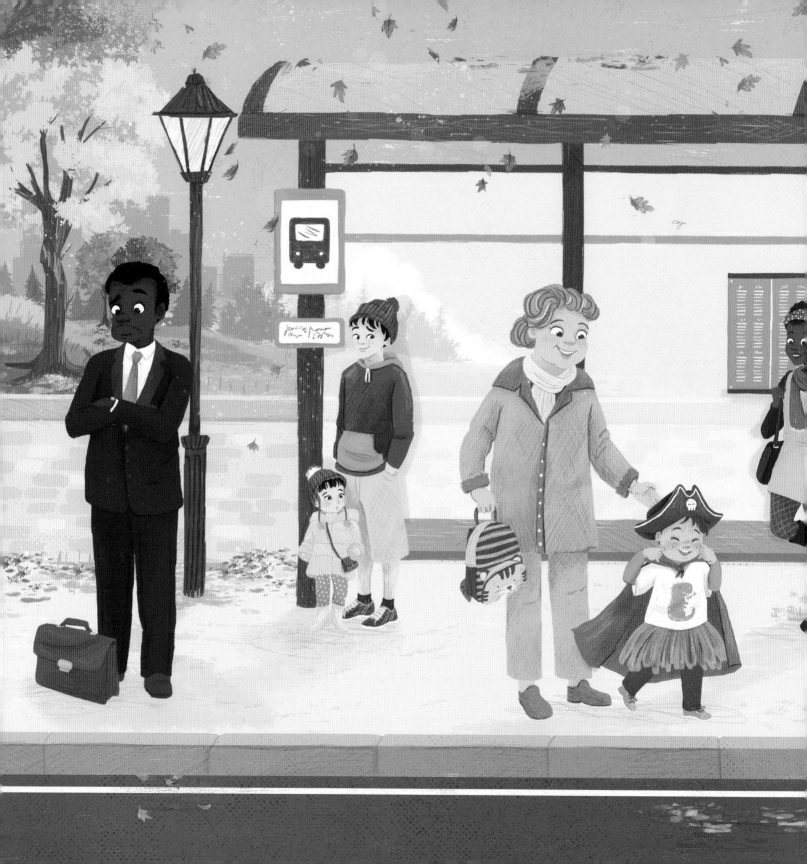

Try to be **GOOD** and **BRAVE** and **STRONG**.

Let people see the real you!

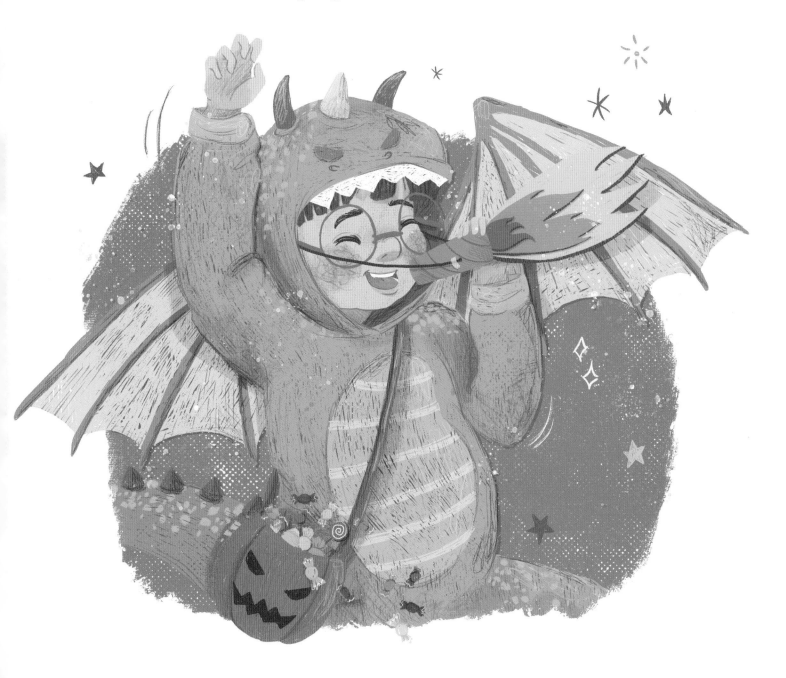

Sometimes things might seem bigger than you.

But you are stronger than your fears.

That's why you have courage.

Courage is when something is scary,
but you do it anyway.

Don't let anyone try to stop you

from taking a chance or trying something new.

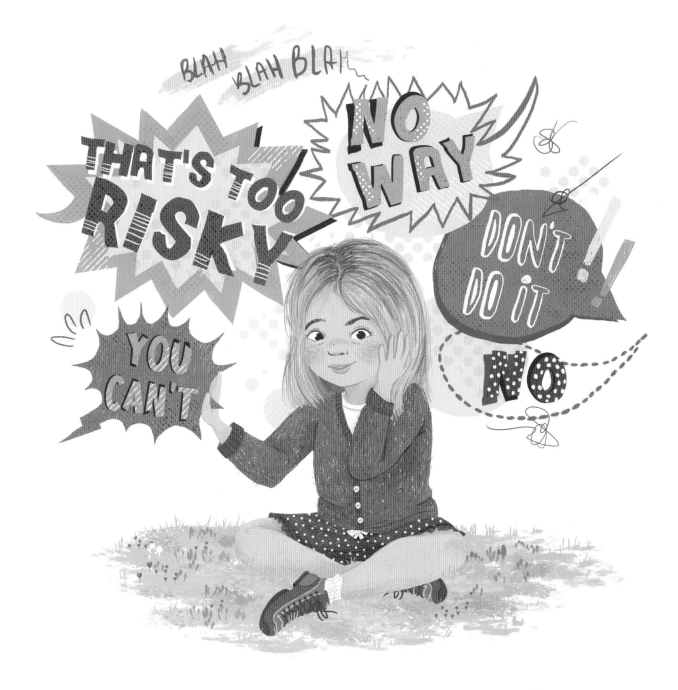

Surround yourself with people who love you.

They are your cheerleaders!

Listen to them when they say:
"Yes, you can!"

When you fall down, get back up.

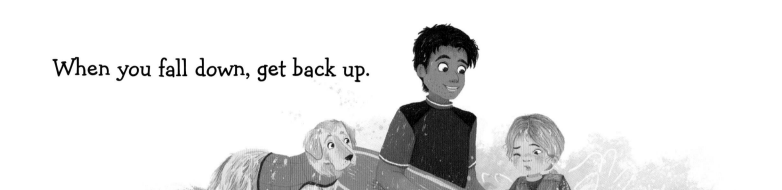

Stay fierce: You know you've got this!

Be YOU wherever you are.

If people stop and stare, just keep going!

Remember, not everyone may understand you.

But that doesn't mean you can't still be happy, just the way that you are.

Never say no to being yourself.

Feel your own beauty, inside and out.

When you let your light shine,

you will brighten the world.

Wouldn't it be boring if
everyone was the same?

Being different is beautiful.

Just **BE YOU**!
Because you are enough.

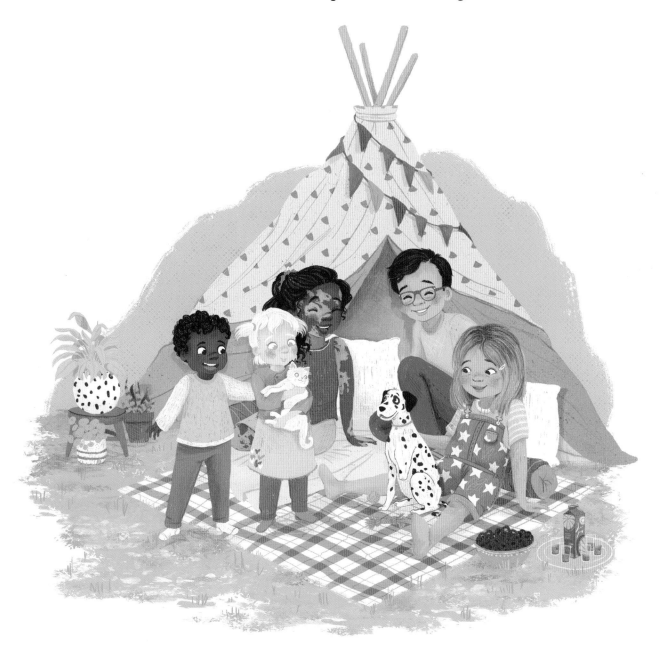

Being enough means you are full of love.

You have purpose.

You aren't perfect
(no one is!).

But you are okay being
perfectly yourself.

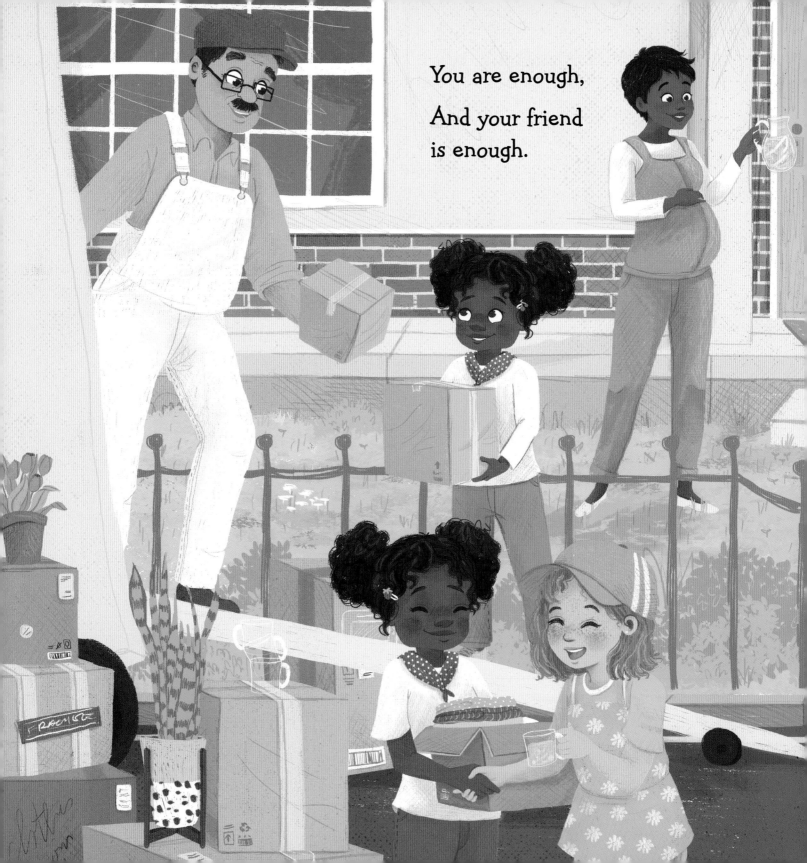

You are enough,
And your friend
is enough.

Your teacher and neighbor are enough, too!

Remember that we all belong.

Look for the good in the world.

Start by looking in the mirror.

Love what you see there.

Because just like me . . .

YOU ARE enough!

ABOUT
SOFIA SANCHEZ

SOFIA SANCHEZ was born in 2009, and she spent the first sixteen months of her life in an orphanage in a small town in Ukraine. In 2010, her parents, Jennifer and Hector Sanchez, adopted her through the organization Reece's Rainbow. Sofia moved to Rocklin, California, where she now lives with her parents and older brothers Diego, Mateo, and Joaquin, who also has Down syndrome. The family has two dogs, Rocco and Lulu, and a cat named Olivia.

In October 2016, Sofia's mom filmed a series of videos of Sofia talking joyfully about what it's like to have Down syndrome. Jennifer posted the videos online in celebration of Down Syndrome Awareness Month, and they quickly went viral. Sofia went on to appear on *CBS Evening News*, *ABC World News Tonight*, *Today*, Univision, and FOX News. She was also featured in *People*, the *Daily Mail UK*, and *USA Today*.

Sofia's career quickly took off, and today she is a model, actress, and an advocate for those with Down syndrome. She has appeared on the Freeform show *Switched at Birth* and in advertisements for Target, Walmart, Hallmark, Pottery Barn, American Girl, Build-a-Bear, and more. Sofia is the star of two previous picture books by author Margaret O'Hair: *Be-You-Tiful: Love, Sofia* tells the true story of Sofia's life, and *Ride the Wave: Love Sofia and Haole the Surf Dog* chronicles Sofia's experience learning to surf with A Walk on Water (AWOW), a non-profit organization that provides surf therapy to children with special needs.

Sofia attends her local public school, where she is fully included in the classroom. Her hobbies include ballet, singing, dancing, swimming, running, gymnastics, and reading. Sofia loves meeting new people and making new friends. She spreads love, joy, and kindness wherever she goes. Sofia understands that her disability does not define her, and her goal is to inspire others to celebrate all the ways they are different and wonderfully themselves.

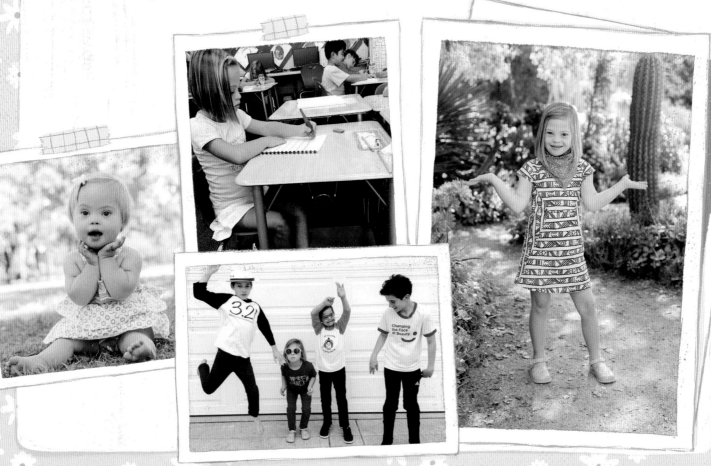

Q&A FOR KiDS FROM THE NATiONAL DoWN SYNDROME SOCiETY

WHAT IS DOWN SYNDROME?

There are trillions of cells in the human body. They are so tiny you can only see them through a microscope. Inside these tiny cells are even tinier parts called chromosomes. Most people have 46 chromosomes in each of their cells. People with Down syndrome have 47 chromosomes instead, and because of that they may look and learn differently.

HOW DO PEOPLE GET DOWN SYNDROME?

People who have Down syndrome are born with it and will always have it. Down syndrome affects both boys and girls all over the world. About one in every 700 babies born in the United States has Down syndrome.

DO KIDS WITH DOWN SYNDROME LIKE THE SAME THINGS AS OTHER KIDS?

Yes! When you get to know someone with Down syndrome, you will find that they have unique personalities and interests, just like everyone else! If they want to, they can play on sports teams, make art, learn to play an instrument, and join clubs at school. They want to have fun and make new friends, like all kids do. People with Down syndrome have feelings. Like all people, they can feel hurt and upset by someone who is mean to them.

TALKING ABOUT DOWN SYNDROME

It is important for people with Down syndrome to be included and supported. Here are some guidelines from the National Down Syndrome Society (NDSS) on the best ways to talk about those with Down syndrome:

- Refer to those with Down syndrome as people first. For example, say "a child with Down syndrome," not "a Down syndrome child."
- Down syndrome is a condition, not a disease. The correct spelling is "Down syndrome," not "Down's syndrome." Avoid calling someone a "Down's child" or "a child with Down's."
- Use the phrase, "She has Down syndrome." Avoid phrases like, "She suffers from Down syndrome," or "She is afflicted by Down syndrome."
- Those without Down syndrome should be referred to as "typical" or "typically developing" rather than "normal."
- Use the phrases "intellectual disability" or "cognitive difference" when talking about Down syndrome.

To learn more about talking to your kids about Down syndrome, visit WWW.NDSS.ORG

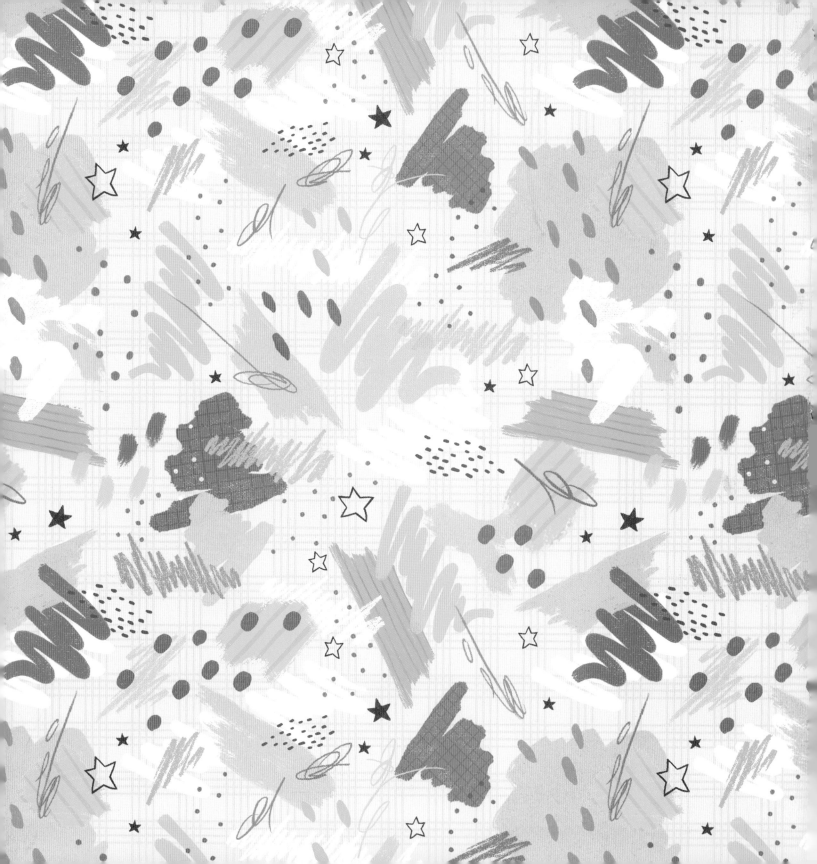